Sugar Free Symphony:

Delicious Delights for a Healthy Blood Sugar Lifestyle

Clifford D. Mason

Table of content

Introduction

Welcome to the vibrant world of Sugar Free Symphony: Delicious Delights for a Healthy Blood Sugar Lifestyle. In a time where our fast-paced lives often lead us to make unhealthy choices, it's imperative to prioritize our well-being and take control of our dietary habits. This book is a harmonious fusion of taste, health, and creativity, designed to guide you on a remarkable journey towards a sugar-free lifestyle that doesn't compromise on flavor or enjoyment.

In the symphony of life, our bodies are the instruments, and the food we consume is the melody. Just like a symphony, each ingredient plays a crucial role, contributing its unique notes to create a beautiful composition. In Sugar Free Symphony, we embrace the idea that a healthy blood sugar lifestyle doesn't have to be bland or monotonous. Instead, it can be a symphony of flavors, colors, and textures, awakening your taste buds while nurturing your body from within.

This book is the result of extensive research, culinary expertise, and a passion for promoting well-being. Its purpose is to empower you with the knowledge and tools needed to make conscious choices about what you eat, without sacrificing the joy of eating. Whether you are managing diabetes, seeking to reduce your sugar intake, or simply striving for a healthier lifestyle, this comprehensive guide will be your trusted companion.

Inside the pages of Sugar Free Symphony, you'll embark on a culinary adventure like no other. From the first chapter to the last, you'll explore a diverse repertoire of delectable recipes that showcase the versatility of sugar-free cooking. Drawing inspiration from global cuisines, traditional favorites, and innovative culinary techniques, these recipes will prove that healthy eating is anything but boring.

Each recipe has been carefully crafted to be low in added sugars, relying instead on natural sweeteners and wholesome ingredients. By focusing on nutrient-dense foods, we can ensure that our bodies receive the essential vitamins, minerals, and fiber they need to thrive. From hearty breakfasts and vibrant salads to soul-warming soups, mouthwatering mains, and guilt-free desserts, every dish in this book celebrates the abundant flavors of nature.

But Sugar Free Symphony is more than just a collection of recipes. It's a comprehensive guide that goes beyond the kitchen. Throughout the book, you'll find valuable insights into the science of blood sugar regulation, the impact of sugar on our health, and practical tips for adopting a sustainable sugar-free lifestyle. We will debunk common myths, address common challenges, and equip you with the knowledge to make informed choices for yourself and your loved ones.

Prepare to be inspired, educated, and delighted as you embark on this transformative culinary journey. Let the symphony of flavors guide you to a healthier and more vibrant way of life. May this book serve as your trusted conductor, helping you orchestrate a delicious, sugar-free symphony that harmonizes your taste buds, nourishes your body, and leads you towards a more fulfilling, vibrant, and sustainable future.

So, grab your apron, tune in to the melody of health, and let Sugar Free Symphony be your guiding light on this extraordinary gastronomic adventure. Your taste buds, body, and overall well-being will thank you. Let the symphony begin!

Chapter 1

About the Blood Sugar Diet

The term "blood sugar diet" refers to a way of eating that focuses on managing and stabilizing blood sugar levels. It is particularly beneficial for individuals with conditions like diabetes or prediabetes, where maintaining stable blood sugar levels is crucial for overall health.

The primary goal of a blood sugar diet is to regulate the amount of glucose (sugar) in the bloodstream, preventing sharp spikes or drops in blood sugar levels. Consistently high blood sugar levels can lead to various health complications, while low blood sugar levels can cause symptoms like fatigue, dizziness, and confusion.

Here are some key principles and strategies commonly associated with a blood sugar diet:

Carbohydrate Management: Carbohydrates have the most significant impact on blood sugar levels. The diet typically involves controlling the amount and type of carbohydrates consumed. Complex carbohydrates with a low glycemic index (GI), such as whole grains, legumes, and non-starchy vegetables, are favored over simple carbohydrates like sugary foods and refined grains.

Portion Control: Managing portion sizes is crucial to prevent excessive carbohydrate intake. Balancing carbohydrate intake with proteins, healthy fats, and fiber-rich foods can help slow down the absorption of glucose and prevent sudden blood sugar spikes.

Glycemic Index (GI): The glycemic index is a ranking system that measures how quickly carbohydrates in food raise blood sugar levels. Foods with a high GI value (such as white bread and sugary snacks) are typically avoided or consumed in moderation, while foods with a low or moderate GI (such as whole grains, fruits, and vegetables) are preferred.

Fiber Intake: Including high-fiber foods in the diet can help slow down the digestion and absorption of carbohydrates, resulting in a more gradual release of glucose into the bloodstream. Foods like whole grains, fruits, vegetables, and legumes are excellent sources of dietary fiber.

Lean Proteins: Including lean proteins in meals and snacks can help stabilize blood sugar levels. Proteins have a minimal impact on blood sugar and can help promote feelings of fullness, reducing the likelihood of overeating carbohydrates. Sources of lean protein include poultry, fish, tofu, legumes, and low-fat dairy products.

Healthy Fats: Incorporating healthy fats, such as those found in avocados, nuts, seeds, and olive oil, can help slow down digestion and provide a steady release of energy. Healthy fats also contribute to overall satiety and can help regulate appetite.

Regular Meal Timing: Establishing regular meal and snack times can help maintain consistent blood sugar levels throughout the day. Spacing meals evenly and avoiding prolonged periods of fasting or excessive snacking can be beneficial.

Hydration: Staying hydrated is essential for overall health and can support healthy blood sugar levels. Drinking water throughout the day and avoiding sugary beverages is recommended.

Regular Physical Activity: Engaging in regular physical activity can help improve insulin sensitivity and promote better blood sugar control. Combining a blood sugar diet with regular exercise is a highly effective approach to managing blood sugar levels.

It's important to note that individual dietary needs may vary, especially for individuals with specific medical conditions. Consulting with a registered dietitian or healthcare professional who specializes in diabetes or blood sugar management is highly recommended to develop a personalized and comprehensive blood sugar diet plan.

How the Blood Sugar Diet can Help Control Blood Sugar Levels

The Blood Sugar Diet is a dietary approach that focuses on controlling blood sugar levels and improving overall health. It is designed to help individuals with conditions like prediabetes, type 2 diabetes, and obesity manage their blood sugar effectively. The diet primarily emphasizes low-carbohydrate, low-calorie, and nutrient-dense foods, and it has gained popularity for its potential benefits in blood sugar control and weight loss.

Low-carbohydrate approach: The Blood Sugar Diet promotes a low-carbohydrate eating plan, which can be beneficial for blood sugar control. Carbohydrates are broken down into glucose, raising blood sugar levels. By reducing carbohydrate intake, the diet helps prevent rapid spikes in blood sugar, which is particularly important for individuals with diabetes.

Glycemic index/load: The diet incorporates the concept of glycemic index (GI) and glycemic load (GL). GI measures how quickly carbohydrates in foods raise blood sugar levels, while GL considers both the quantity and quality of carbohydrates consumed. The Blood Sugar Diet encourages foods with a low GI and GL, such as non-starchy vegetables, legumes, and whole grains, which have a minimal impact on blood sugar levels.

Calorie restriction: The Blood Sugar Diet also focuses on calorie restriction, which can aid in weight loss and blood sugar control. By reducing overall calorie intake, the diet helps create a calorie deficit, leading to weight loss. Weight loss has been shown to improve insulin sensitivity, allowing better blood sugar regulation.

Nutrient-dense foods: While the diet restricts calories and carbohydrates, it emphasizes nutrient-dense foods. This means that the diet promotes the consumption of foods that are rich in vitamins, minerals, and other essential nutrients. Nutrient-dense foods support overall health, provide satiety, and can help prevent nutrient deficiencies.

Intermittent fasting: The Blood Sugar Diet incorporates intermittent fasting, which involves cycling between periods of fasting and eating. This approach can help control blood sugar levels by allowing the body to better regulate insulin and improve insulin sensitivity. Fasting periods give the body a break from constantly processing food, promoting more stable blood sugar levels.

Weight loss benefits: Excess weight is closely linked to insulin resistance and impaired blood sugar control. The Blood Sugar Diet's emphasis on calorie restriction and nutrient-dense foods can lead to weight loss, reducing the risk of developing type 2 diabetes and improving blood sugar management for those already diagnosed.

Enhanced insulin sensitivity: The Blood Sugar Diet's combination of low-carbohydrate eating, calorie restriction, and intermittent fasting can enhance insulin sensitivity. Improved insulin sensitivity allows the body to utilize insulin more efficiently, leading to better blood sugar control.

It is important to note that while the Blood Sugar Diet can be beneficial for blood sugar control, it should be followed under the guidance of a healthcare professional, especially for individuals with diabetes who may require adjustments to medication dosages. Consulting a registered dietitian or healthcare provider can help tailor the diet to individual needs and ensure adequate nutrition while managing blood sugar levels effectively.

Key Principles of Blood Sugar Diet

The key principles of the Blood Sugar Diet are as follows:

Low-Carbohydrate, Low-Sugar Intake: The diet recommends reducing the consumption of carbohydrates, especially refined carbohydrates and added sugars.

This includes limiting or eliminating foods such as white bread, pasta, sugary beverages, sweets, and processed snacks.

Balanced Macronutrient Ratio: The Blood Sugar Diet encourages a balanced macronutrient ratio, with a moderate intake of protein, healthy fats, and complex carbohydrates from non-starchy vegetables, legumes, and whole grains. This balanced approach helps stabilize blood sugar levels and provides sustained energy.

Low-Glycemic Index Foods: The diet emphasizes consuming low-glycemic index (GI) foods. The GI is a measure of how quickly a particular food raises blood sugar levels. Low-GI foods, such as non-starchy vegetables, nuts, seeds, and berries, are digested more slowly, resulting in a gradual and steady release of glucose into the bloodstream.

Intermittent Fasting: The Blood Sugar Diet incorporates intermittent fasting as a strategy to improve insulin sensitivity and promote weight loss. This involves restricting calorie intake for specific periods, typically by following a time-restricted eating pattern, such as 16:8 (fasting for 16 hours, eating within an 8-hour window).

Adequate Fiber Intake: The diet encourages consuming an adequate amount of dietary fiber, which helps slow down the digestion and absorption of carbohydrates, preventing rapid spikes in blood sugar levels. Fiber-rich foods include whole grains, legumes, fruits, vegetables, and nuts.

Mindful Eating: The Blood Sugar Diet emphasizes mindful eating practices, such as paying attention to hunger and fullness cues, eating slowly, and savoring each bite. This approach promotes better food choices and prevents overeating.

Regular Physical Activity: Exercise is an integral part of the Blood Sugar Diet. Engaging in regular physical activity helps improve insulin sensitivity, promotes weight loss, and supports overall blood sugar control. Both aerobic exercises (e.g., walking, jogging, cycling) and strength training are recommended.

Personalization and Sustainability: The Blood Sugar Diet acknowledges that individual needs and preferences may vary. It encourages personalized meal planning based on one's health goals, body composition, and lifestyle. The diet also promotes long-term sustainability, aiming for a lifestyle change rather than a short-term fix.

Chapter 2: Understanding Blood Sugar

What is Blood Sugar?

Blood sugar, often known as blood glucose, refers to the concentration of glucose (a form of sugar) in the bloodstream. Glucose is the major source of energy for the body's cells, and it plays a critical part in sustaining general physical processes. Blood sugar levels are controlled by a complicated interplay of different hormones, principally insulin and glucagon, generated by the pancreas.

When we ingest carbs (such as grains, fruits, and vegetables), the digestive system breaks them down into glucose. This glucose is subsequently taken into the system, causing blood sugar levels to increase. In reaction to rising blood sugar levels, the pancreas produces insulin, a hormone that helps glucose enter the cells and be used for energy.

Maintaining blood sugar within a limited range is vital for general health and well-being. Very low blood sugar levels (hypoglycemia) may result in symptoms including weakness, disorientation, confusion, and, in severe instances, loss of consciousness. On the other side, consistently high blood sugar levels (hyperglycemia) may lead to diabetes and numerous problems, such as damage to blood vessels, neurons, and organs.

In persons without diabetes, the body's regulatory systems work to maintain blood sugar levels steady. However, in persons with diabetes, this control is disrupted. There are two basic forms of diabetes: type 1 and type 2. In type 1 diabetes, the body does not create enough insulin, needing insulin injections for adequate blood sugar regulation. In type 2 diabetes, the body develops resistant to the effects of insulin or does not generate enough insulin.

Monitoring blood sugar levels is critical for those with diabetes, as it helps them make educated choices regarding medicine, nutrition, and physical exercise. This is frequently done by using a blood glucose meter to assess the glucose concentration in a tiny blood sample, usually acquired by pricking the finger. Continuous glucose monitoring (CGM) devices are also available, which offer real-time blood sugar readings throughout the day.

To maintain normal blood sugar levels, a balanced diet, frequent physical exercise, and suitable medication (if required) are necessary. Diet has a vital impact since carbohydrates directly affect blood sugar levels. Monitoring carbohydrate consumption and preferring complex carbs (e.g., whole grains) over simple sugars (e.g., sugary beverages) will help regulate blood sugar levels efficiently.

The Role of Insulin

Insulin serves a critical function in controlling blood sugar levels in the human body. It is a hormone generated by the pancreas, primarily by beta cells in the islets of Langerhans. The major purpose of insulin is to assist the absorption, use, and storage of glucose (sugar) from the circulation into cells throughout the body. This procedure helps to maintain steady blood sugar levels, which is crucial for general health and normal physical functioning.

When we ingest carbs, such as bread, rice, or fruits, they are broken down into glucose during digestion and absorbed into the circulation. Elevated blood glucose levels prompt the production of insulin from the pancreas. Insulin then interacts to particular receptors on cell surfaces, allowing glucose to enter cells from the circulation.

The function of insulin in blood sugar management may be described via the following mechanisms:

Glucose uptake: Insulin increases the translocation of glucose transporters, specifically GLUT4, to the cell membrane. These transporters promote the entrance of glucose into muscle, fat, and liver cells, where it may be consumed for energy generation or stored for later use.

Glycogen synthesis: In addition to urgent energy demands, surplus glucose may be turned into glycogen, a storage form of glucose. Insulin increases glycogen production (glycogenesis) largely in the liver and muscle cells, therefore avoiding excessive buildup of glucose in the circulation.

Inhibition of gluconeogenesis:
Gluconeogenesis is the process by which the liver manufactures glucose from non-carbohydrate sources, such as amino acids and glycerol. Insulin suppresses gluconeogenesis, lowering the liver's generation of glucose and helping to keep blood sugar levels within a normal range.

Lipid metabolism: Insulin impacts lipid metabolism by boosting the absorption of fatty acids and preventing their release from adipose tissue. It promotes the production of triglycerides (storage form of fats) and decreases the breakdown of stored fats (lipolysis). This process guarantees that glucose is prioritized as an energy source, particularly in the presence of sufficient carbs.

Protein synthesis: Insulin plays a critical function in protein metabolism by boosting amino acid absorption into cells and driving protein synthesis. It aids the development, maintenance, and repair of bodily tissues.

Insulin resistance is a condition in which cells become less sensitive to the actions of insulin. This may lead to high blood sugar levels and, ultimately, type 2 diabetes if left mismanaged. In type 1 diabetes, the body cannot generate insulin, necessitating patients to receive exogenous insulin to maintain their blood sugar levels.

Maintaining normal blood sugar levels is vital for general health. If blood sugar levels are continually excessively high (hyperglycemia), it may lead to long-term issues, such as cardiovascular disease, renal damage, nerve damage, and eye difficulties. On the other side, if blood sugar levels are regularly excessively low (hypoglycemia), it may induce symptoms including weakness, disorientation, dizziness, and, in extreme instances, loss of consciousness.

Impact of High and Low Blood Sugar Levels

High and low blood sugar levels may have substantial consequences on the body and overall health. Maintaining steady blood sugar levels is vital for the efficient functioning of different body systems. Let's explore the effect of high and low blood sugar levels in detail:

Impact of High Blood Sugar
(Hyperglycemia): High blood sugar arises when the body fails to generate enough insulin or adequately use insulin, resulting to an excess of glucose in the bloodstream. The consequence of persistent high blood sugar levels includes:
a. Diabetes complications: Prolonged hyperglycemia may result in different complications linked with diabetes, such as cardiovascular illness, kidney damage, nerve damage (neuropathy), eye issues (retinopathy), and sluggish wound healing.

b. Diabetic ketoacidosis (DKA): Extremely high blood sugar levels may precipitate a disease termed DKA, most typically observed in persons with type 1 diabetes. It is a potentially life-threatening disorder characterized by the formation of ketones and acidity of the blood.

c. Dehydration: High blood sugar produces increased urine, leading to fluid loss and dehydration. This might result in symptoms including increased thirst, dry mouth, and weariness.

d. Increased risk of infections: Hyperglycemia impairs the immune system, making persons more prone to infections, notably urinary tract infections, yeast infections, and skin infections.

e. Cardiovascular problems: Elevated blood sugar levels may damage blood arteries, leading to an increased risk of heart disease, heart attack, and stroke.

f. Nerve damage: High blood sugar may cause damage to the nerves, resulting in symptoms such as numbness, tingling, and burning sensations in the extremities.

Impact of Low Blood Sugar (Hypoglycemia): Low blood sugar develops when there is an insufficient amount of glucose in the circulation. It is usually related with diabetic treatments, notably insulin. The effect of low blood sugar levels includes:
a. Neurological symptoms: Hypoglycemia impairs brain function, resulting to symptoms including disorientation, dizziness, trouble focusing, and even seizures or loss of consciousness if severe.

b. exhaustion and weakness: Low blood sugar levels may produce a lack of energy, exhaustion, and weakness, making it difficult to accomplish everyday tasks.

c. Emotional disturbances: Hypoglycemia may produce mood swings, impatience, anxiety, and even depressed symptoms.

d. accelerated heart rate: The body produces stress chemicals, such as adrenaline, in reaction to low blood sugar, resulting in an accelerated heart rate and palpitations.

a. Impaired cognitive function: When the brain is deprived of glucose, cognitive functions such as memory, problem-solving, and coordination might be severely affected.

f. Potential accidents: Severe hypoglycemia may lead to disorientation or loss of consciousness, raising the risk of accidents or injuries, particularly while using equipment or driving.

Managing blood sugar levels within a healthy range is critical for those with diabetes or those at risk of developing diabetes. This often entails lifestyle adjustments, including a balanced diet, frequent exercise, correct medication (if required), and regular blood sugar testing.

It is vital for persons with diabetes to work closely with healthcare providers to build a personalized strategy for controlling blood sugar levels successfully and avoiding the risk of problems associated with high or low blood sugar.

Importance of Balancing Blood Sugar for Overall Health

Balancing blood sugar levels is vital for preserving general health and well-being. Here are some basic reasons why regulating blood sugar is vital for general health:

Diabetes Management: Blood sugar homeostasis is especially crucial for those with diabetes. Diabetes is a chronic illness characterized by excessive blood sugar levels. Proper blood sugar control via food, exercise, medication, and monitoring may help patients with diabetes avoid consequences such as heart disease, kidney damage, nerve damage, and eye difficulties.

Energy Regulation: Balanced blood sugar levels are crucial for giving a consistent supply of energy to the body's cells. Glucose is the major source of energy for the body, and maintaining constant blood sugar levels maintains a steady energy supply. When blood sugar levels are unbalanced, it might result in weariness, lethargy, and difficulties focusing.

Weight Management: Blood sugar imbalance may lead to weight gain and obesity. When blood sugar levels climb, the body produces insulin to help transport glucose into the cells. Excessive insulin production might encourage fat accumulation and contribute to weight gain. Additionally, uneven blood sugar might trigger desires for sweet and high-calorie meals, making it tougher to maintain a healthy weight.

Cardiovascular Health: Elevated blood sugar levels, especially in persons with diabetes, may dramatically raise the risk of cardiovascular disorders such as heart disease and stroke. Uncontrolled blood sugar may damage blood vessels and hamper circulation, leading to atherosclerosis (hardening of the arteries) and other cardiovascular issues. Balancing blood sugar helps lower the risk of these illnesses and enhances cardiovascular health.

Mental Health: Research reveals a substantial relationship between blood sugar levels and mental health. Fluctuations in blood sugar may impair mood, cognition, and general mental well-being. Low blood sugar (hypoglycemia) may induce irritation, disorientation, and trouble focusing. On the other side, high blood sugar (hyperglycemia) has been connected with symptoms such as weariness, anxiety, and sadness. By keeping normal blood sugar levels, people may promote their mental health.

Hormonal Balance: Blood sugar abnormalities may alter the delicate balance of hormones in the body. Insulin resistance, a disease where cells become less receptive to the actions of insulin, is commonly accompanied with hormonal abnormalities, especially in women. These abnormalities may influence menstrual cycles, fertility, and general hormone homeostasis. By regulating blood sugar levels, people may maintain hormonal equilibrium.

Long-Term Health: Consistently elevated blood sugar levels over time may contribute to the development of chronic illnesses such as type 2 diabetes, metabolic syndrome, and insulin resistance. These disorders are related with an increased risk of many health issues, including heart disease, stroke, kidney disease, nerve damage, and eye impairment. Balancing blood sugar may help avoid the emergence of certain long-term health concerns.

Chapter 3: Getting Started with the Blood Sugar Diet

Preparing Your Kitchen for Success

Preparing your kitchen for success is crucial when following the blood sugar diet. This dietary approach focuses on stabilizing blood sugar levels and promoting weight loss by reducing carbohydrate intake and incorporating healthy fats and proteins. By setting up your kitchen to support this lifestyle, you can make it easier to stick to the diet and achieve your health goals. Here are some tips for preparing your kitchen for success on the blood sugar diet:

Clear Out Unhealthy Foods: Start by removing sugary snacks, processed foods, refined grains, sugary beverages, and unhealthy fats from your pantry and refrigerator. These items can spike your blood sugar levels and hinder your progress.

Instead, stock your kitchen with fresh, whole foods.

Stock Up on Healthy Foods: Fill your kitchen with a variety of nutrient-dense foods that support the blood sugar diet. This includes fresh vegetables (leafy greens, broccoli, cauliflower, bell peppers), lean proteins (chicken, turkey, fish, tofu), healthy fats (avocados, nuts, seeds, olive oil), and low-sugar fruits (berries, apples, citrus fruits).

Plan and Prep Meals: Meal planning and prepping can save you time and help you make healthier choices. Set aside time each week to plan your meals and create a shopping list. Consider batch cooking and portioning meals in advance to have healthy options readily available. This reduces the likelihood of reaching for unhealthy convenience foods.

Use Low-Carb Substitutes: Look for low-carb alternatives to common high-carb ingredients. For example, use cauliflower rice or zucchini noodles instead of white rice or pasta. Use lettuce wraps or collard greens instead of tortillas or bread for sandwiches and wraps. Experiment with almond flour or coconut flour as substitutes for regular flour in baking.

Invest in Quality Cooking Tools: Having the right cooking tools can make preparing healthy meals easier and more enjoyable. Consider investing in a good set of knives, a quality blender or food processor, a steamer, and non-stick cookware. These tools will help you prepare a variety of dishes and make cooking more efficient.

Organize Your Kitchen: Keep your kitchen organized to minimize stress and confusion. Arrange your pantry with healthy staples at eye level, making them more accessible. Store spices and herbs in a designated area for easy access. Keep your refrigerator and freezer organized with clearly labeled containers to avoid wasting food and make meal prep more efficient.

Read Food Labels: Develop the habit of reading food labels to make informed choices. Look for foods that are low in added sugars, refined grains, and unhealthy fats. Pay attention to serving sizes and carbohydrate content, especially if you're monitoring your blood sugar levels closely.

Stay Hydrated: Keep a water pitcher or a bottle within reach in your kitchen to remind you to stay hydrated throughout the day. Drinking enough water helps control appetite and maintain proper hydration, which is essential for overall health and wellbeing.

Incorporate Herbs and Spices: Experiment with herbs and spices to add flavor to your meals without relying on excessive salt, sugar, or unhealthy sauces. Cinnamon, turmeric, garlic, ginger, and cayenne pepper are just a few examples of flavorful ingredients that can enhance your dishes and provide potential health benefits.

Seek Support: Consider involving your family or household members in the blood sugar diet. Support from loved ones can help you stay motivated and make healthier choices together. Encourage open communication about your goals and educate them about the benefits of the blood sugar diet.

Stocking Up on Blood Sugar-Friendly Ingredients

Stocking up on blood sugar-friendly ingredients is an important step for individuals looking to manage or prevent conditions such as diabetes, hypoglycemia, or insulin resistance. By carefully selecting the right foods, you can help regulate blood sugar levels and promote overall health. We will explore the concept of blood sugar-friendly ingredients, provide examples of such ingredients, and offer tips for incorporating them into your diet.

Understanding blood sugar-friendly ingredients:
Blood sugar-friendly ingredients are foods that have a minimal impact on blood sugar levels or help regulate them. They typically have a low glycemic index (GI) or contain nutrients that slow down the absorption of glucose into the bloodstream. These ingredients can help prevent blood sugar spikes, promote stable energy levels, and support overall metabolic health.

Examples of blood sugar-friendly ingredients:
a. Non-starchy vegetables: Leafy greens, broccoli, cauliflower, zucchini, and peppers are excellent choices as they are low in

carbohydrates and high in fiber, which aids in slowing down the release of glucose into the bloodstream.

b. Whole grains: Opt for whole grains such as quinoa, brown rice, barley, and whole wheat bread instead of refined grains. They contain more fiber and have a lower GI, making them a better choice for managing blood sugar.

c. Legumes: Beans, lentils, and chickpeas are rich in fiber, protein, and complex carbohydrates. They provide a gradual release of glucose, preventing blood sugar spikes.

d. Lean proteins: Incorporating lean sources of protein like skinless poultry, fish, tofu, and eggs in your diet can help regulate blood sugar levels and promote satiety.

e. Healthy fats: Include foods rich in healthy fats, such as avocados, nuts, seeds, and olive oil. They help slow down the digestion of carbohydrates and promote stable blood sugar levels.

f. Berries: Berries like strawberries, blueberries, and raspberries are low in sugar and high in fiber, antioxidants, and other beneficial compounds. They have a lower impact on blood sugar compared to other fruits.

g. Cinnamon: This spice has been shown to help improve insulin sensitivity and regulate blood sugar levels. It can be added to various dishes or beverages.

h. Vinegar: Consuming vinegar, such as apple cider vinegar, with meals has been found to improve insulin sensitivity and lower post-meal blood sugar levels.

Tips for incorporating blood sugar-friendly ingredients into your diet:

a. Plan your meals: Create a meal plan that includes a balance of blood sugar-friendly ingredients, focusing on lean proteins, non-starchy vegetables, whole grains, and healthy fats.

b. Read food labels: When grocery shopping, check the nutritional information and ingredient lists. Look for products that are low in added sugars, high in fiber, and made with whole food ingredients.

c. Control portion sizes: Even blood sugar-friendly foods should be consumed in moderation. Pay attention to portion sizes to avoid overeating and maintain stable blood sugar levels.

d. Cook at home: Preparing meals at home gives you better control over the ingredients you use. Experiment with recipes that incorporate blood sugar-friendly ingredients.

e. Snack wisely: Choose healthy snacks like raw vegetables with hummus, a handful of nuts, or Greek yogurt with berries to keep your blood sugar stable between meals.

f. Stay hydrated: Drinking water throughout the day helps maintain hydration and can help prevent overeating or cravings for sugary foods.

g. Monitor your blood sugar levels: If you have specific health concerns related to blood sugar, it's important to monitor your levels regularly. Consult with a healthcare professional for personalized guidance and to make any necessary adjustments to your diet or treatment plan.

Planning Your Meals and Snacks

Planning your meals and snacks is essential when following a blood sugar diet. This type of diet focuses on managing blood glucose levels to prevent spikes and maintain stable insulin response. By carefully selecting nutritious foods, controlling portion sizes, and incorporating balanced meals and snacks, you can help regulate blood sugar levels and improve overall health.

Understand the basics of a blood sugar diet:

A blood sugar diet emphasizes consuming complex carbohydrates with a low glycemic index (GI). These carbs are digested and absorbed slowly, causing a gradual rise in blood sugar levels.

It involves incorporating lean proteins, healthy fats, fiber-rich foods, and a variety of vegetables into your meals.

Avoid or limit foods that are high in added sugars, refined grains, unhealthy fats, and processed ingredients.

Consult with a healthcare professional or a registered dietitian: Before embarking on any dietary changes, it is important to consult a healthcare professional or a registered dietitian to get personalized guidance and ensure the diet suits your specific needs.

Plan balanced meals:
Include a combination of complex carbohydrates, lean proteins, and healthy fats in each meal.
Complex carbohydrates: Choose whole grains such as quinoa, brown rice, whole wheat bread, and oats. These provide fiber and nutrients while minimizing blood sugar spikes.

Lean proteins: Opt for sources like skinless poultry, fish, legumes, tofu, and low-fat dairy products. Proteins help stabilize blood sugar levels and provide satiety.

Healthy fats: Include sources like avocados, nuts, seeds, olive oil, and fatty fish. These fats are beneficial for heart health and aid in blood sugar control.

Vegetables: Aim for a variety of non-starchy vegetables like leafy greens, broccoli, cauliflower, bell peppers, and tomatoes. These are low in calories and high in fiber and nutrients.

Choose appropriate snacks:
Snacks are an important part of a blood sugar diet to prevent hunger and maintain steady blood glucose levels.
Opt for snacks that combine protein, healthy fats, and fiber-rich carbohydrates.
Examples of blood sugar-friendly snacks include a handful of nuts, Greek yogurt with berries, carrot sticks with hummus, apple slices with almond butter, or a small portion of whole grain crackers with cottage cheese.

Monitor portion sizes:
Portion control is crucial for managing blood sugar levels and overall calorie intake. Use measuring cups, food scales, or visual cues to estimate appropriate portion sizes. Focus on consuming balanced portions of each food group to ensure a well-rounded meal.

Include fiber-rich foods:
Fiber helps slow down the absorption of glucose, preventing blood sugar spikes. Incorporate whole grains, legumes, fruits, vegetables, and seeds in your meals and snacks to boost fiber intake.

Stay hydrated:
Water plays a vital role in maintaining overall health and managing blood sugar levels.
Drink an adequate amount of water throughout the day and limit sugary beverages like soda, fruit juices, and energy drinks.

Meal prep and planning:
Plan your meals and snacks in advance to avoid impulsive food choices.
Consider meal prepping by cooking larger batches of meals and portioning them for future consumption. This helps in maintaining consistency and saves time during busy days.

Regular monitoring and adjustments:
Continuously monitor your blood sugar levels and work with your healthcare team to make any necessary adjustments to your diet and medication.
Everyone's body responds differently, so it's important to track how different foods and meal timings affect your blood glucose levels.

Chapter 4: Breakfast and Brunch Recipes

Energizing Breakfast Smoothie

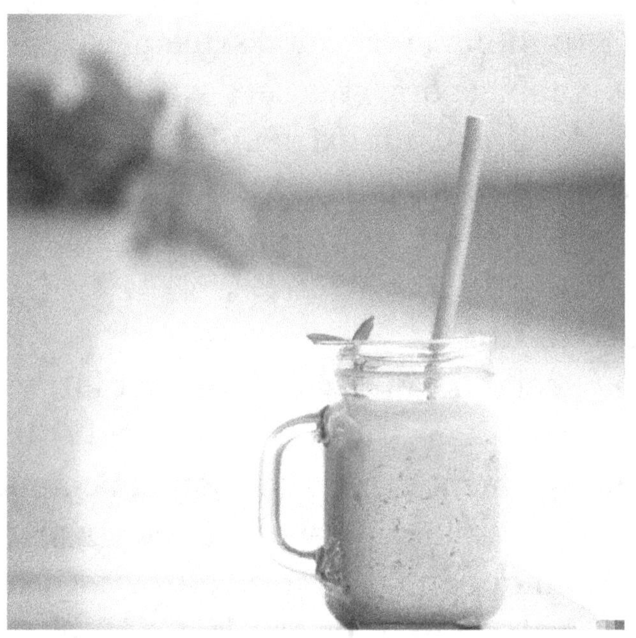

Ingredients:
- 1 ripe banana
- 1 cup fresh spinach leaves
- 1/2 cup plain Greek yogurt

- 1/2 cup almond milk (or any other milk of your choice)
- 1 tablespoon almond butter or peanut butter
- 1 tablespoon honey or maple syrup (optional, for added sweetness)
- 1 tablespoon chia seeds or flaxseeds (optional, for extra nutrition)
- Ice cubes (optional, for a colder smoothie)

Instructions:
- Peel the banana and break it into chunks.
- In a blender, add the banana chunks, fresh spinach leaves, Greek yogurt, almond milk, almond butter or peanut butter, honey or maple syrup (if using), and chia seeds or flaxseeds (if using).
- Blend the ingredients until smooth and creamy. If you prefer a colder smoothie, you can add a few ice cubes

and blend again until the desired consistency is reached.
- Taste the smoothie and adjust the sweetness if needed by adding more honey or maple syrup.
- Once you're satisfied with the taste and texture, pour the smoothie into a glass and enjoy it immediately.

This energizing breakfast smoothie is packed with nutrients from the spinach, banana, Greek yogurt, and nut butter. It provides a good balance of carbohydrates, protein, and healthy fats to fuel your morning and keep you energized throughout the day. Feel free to customize the recipe by adding other fruits, such as berries or mango, or by incorporating your favorite superfoods like spirulina or maca powder.

Vegetable and Egg Scramble

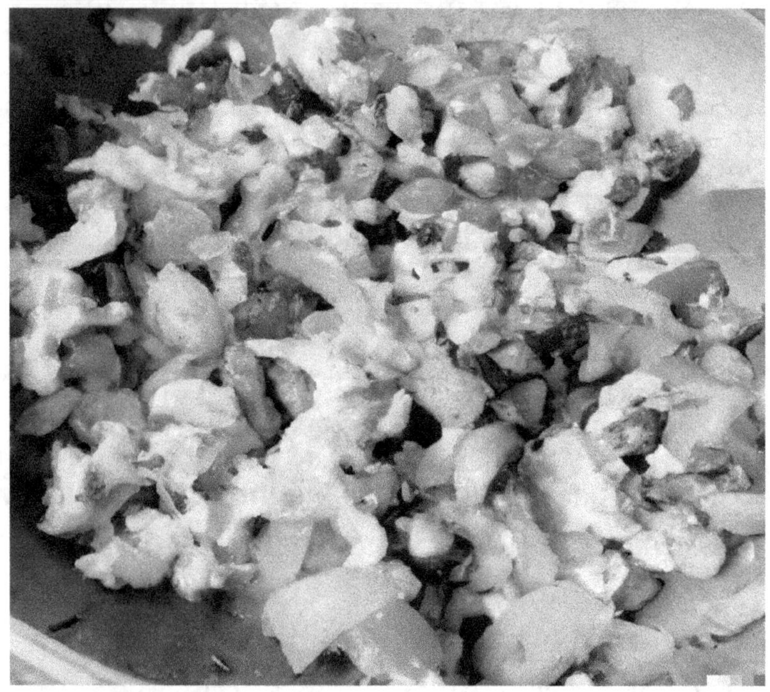

Ingredients:

- 2 tablespoons oil (olive oil, vegetable oil, or your preferred cooking oil)
- 1 small onion, diced
- 1 bell pepper, diced
- 1 zucchini, diced
- 1 cup sliced mushrooms

- 4-6 eggs
- Salt and pepper to taste
- Optional toppings: grated cheese, chopped fresh herbs (such as parsley or chives)

Instructions:

- Heat the oil in a large skillet or frying pan over medium heat.
- Add the diced onion and bell pepper to the pan and sauté for about 3-4 minutes, until they start to soften.
- Add the diced zucchini and sliced mushrooms to the pan and continue cooking for another 3-4 minutes, until the vegetables are tender.
- While the vegetables are cooking, crack the eggs into a bowl and whisk them together. Season with salt and pepper.
- Pour the beaten eggs into the pan with the cooked vegetables. Stir gently to combine everything.

- Cook the mixture, stirring occasionally, until the eggs are cooked to your desired doneness. If you prefer a more well-done scramble, cook for a few minutes longer.
- Once the eggs are cooked, remove the pan from the heat.
- Sprinkle grated cheese and chopped fresh herbs on top, if desired.
- Serve the vegetable and egg scramble hot as a delicious and nutritious breakfast or brunch option.

Feel free to customize the recipe by adding or substituting vegetables based on your preferences. Enjoy your meal!

Almond Flour Pancakes

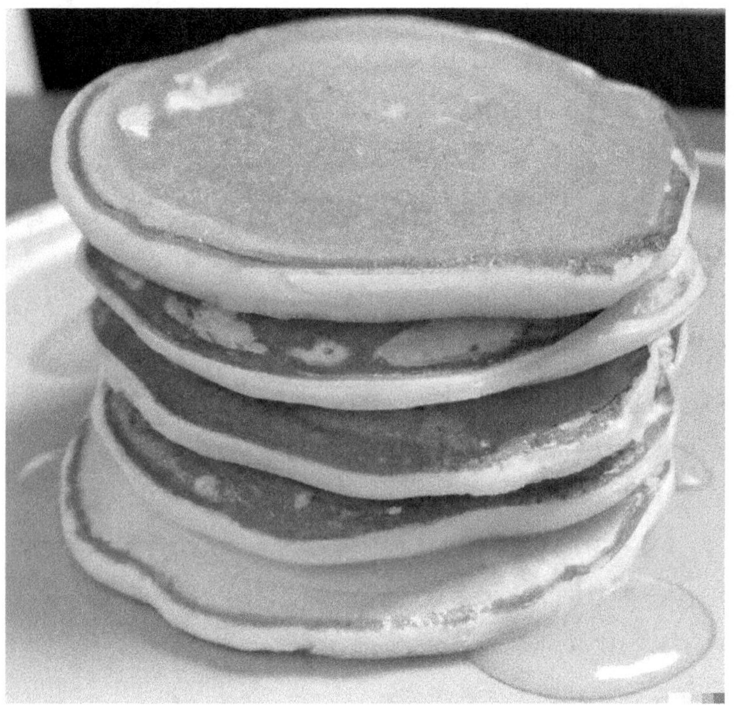

Ingredients:

- 1 cup almond flour
- 2 tablespoons coconut flour
- 2 tablespoons sweetener of your choice (e.g., honey, maple syrup, or stevia)

- 1/2 teaspoon baking powder
- 1/4 teaspoon salt
- 4 large eggs
- 1/2 cup milk (dairy or non-dairy)
- 1 teaspoon vanilla extract
- Coconut oil or butter for cooking

Instructions:
In a mixing bowl, combine the almond flour, coconut flour, sweetener, baking powder, and salt. Mix well to ensure all the ingredients are evenly distributed.

In a separate bowl, whisk together the eggs, milk, and vanilla extract until well combined.

Pour the wet ingredients into the dry ingredients and stir until a smooth batter forms. Let the batter sit for a few minutes to allow the flours to absorb the liquid.

Heat a non-stick skillet or griddle over
medium heat and add a small amount of
coconut oil or butter to coat the surface.

Scoop about 1/4 cup of batter onto the
skillet for each pancake. Use the back of a
spoon to spread the batter into a circular
shape if needed. Cook for 2-3 minutes, or
until bubbles form on the surface.

Flip the pancakes using a spatula and cook
for an additional 1-2 minutes, or until
golden brown and cooked through.

Remove the pancakes from the skillet and
repeat the process with the remaining
batter, adding more oil or butter to the
skillet as needed.

Serve the almond flour pancakes warm with
your favorite toppings such as fresh berries,
sliced bananas, nut butter, or a drizzle of
maple syrup.

Chia Seed Pudding

Chia seed pudding is a popular and nutritious dish made with chia seeds and a liquid of your choice. Chia seeds are small, black seeds that come from the Salvia hispanica plant, native to Mexico. They are packed with nutrients like omega-3 fatty acids, fiber, protein, and various minerals.

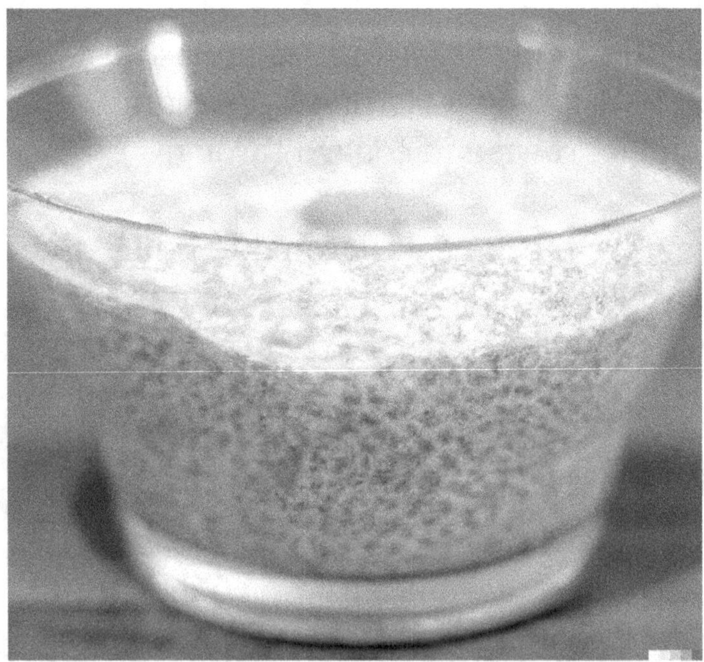

To make chia seed pudding, you'll need the following ingredients:

- 1/4 cup chia seeds
- 1 cup liquid (such as almond milk, coconut milk, or regular milk)
- Sweetener of your choice (honey, maple syrup, or sugar)
- Flavorings (vanilla extract, cocoa powder, fruit, etc., optional)
- Toppings (fruit, nuts, coconut flakes, etc., optional)

Here's a simple recipe to make chia seed pudding:

In a bowl or container, combine the chia seeds and liquid. Stir well to ensure the chia seeds are evenly distributed.

Add sweetener to taste. Start with about 1-2 tablespoons and adjust according to your preference. You can also add flavorings like vanilla extract, cocoa powder, or mashed fruit at this stage if desired.

Stir the mixture thoroughly until the chia seeds are well coated. This helps prevent clumping.

Let the mixture sit for about 5 minutes and then stir again to break up any clumps that may have formed.

Cover the bowl or container and refrigerate for at least 2 hours or overnight. During this time, the chia seeds will absorb the liquid and turn into a pudding-like consistency.

Before serving, give the pudding a good stir to distribute any settled chia seeds. If the pudding appears too thick, you can add a little more liquid to achieve your desired consistency.

Serve the chia seed pudding chilled and garnish with your favorite toppings such as fresh fruits, nuts, or coconut flakes.

Chia seed pudding can be enjoyed as a healthy breakfast, snack, or even as a dessert. It's a versatile dish, and you can experiment with different flavors and toppings to suit your taste preferences.

Mediterranean Omelet

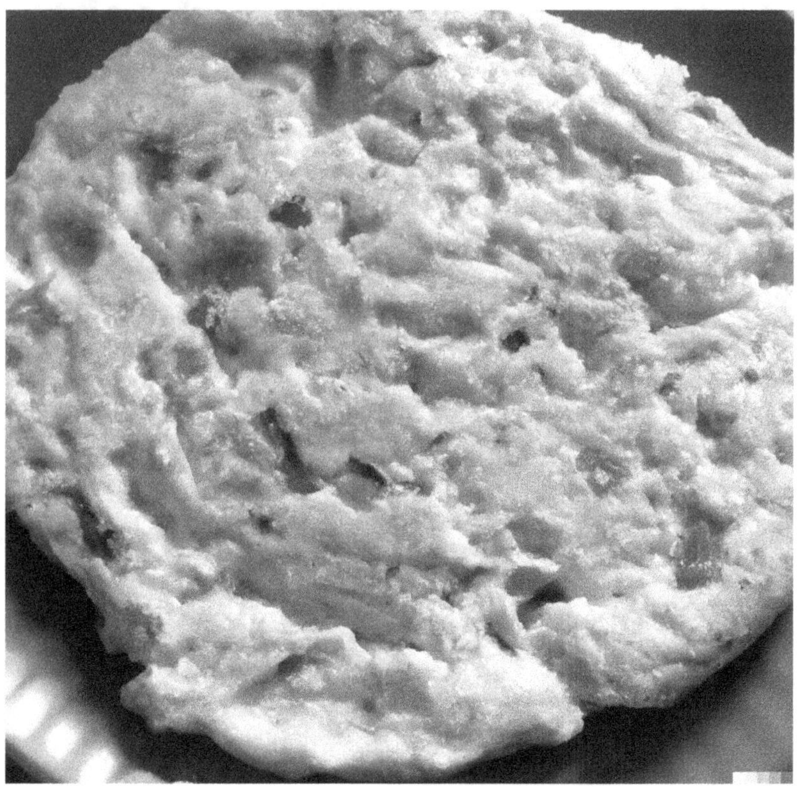

Ingredients:

- 3 large eggs
- 2 tablespoons olive oil
- 1/4 cup diced red bell pepper
- 1/4 cup diced red onion
- 1/4 cup sliced black olives
- 1/4 cup chopped fresh spinach
- 1/4 cup crumbled feta cheese
- 2 tablespoons chopped fresh parsley
- Salt and pepper to taste

Instructions:

- Crack the eggs into a bowl and beat them lightly with a fork or whisk. Season with salt and pepper according to your taste.
- Heat 1 tablespoon of olive oil in a non-stick skillet over medium heat.
- Add the diced red bell pepper and red onion to the skillet and sauté for about 2-3 minutes until they start to soften.
- Add the sliced black olives and chopped spinach to the skillet and

cook for another minute until the spinach wilts.

- Remove the vegetables from the skillet and set aside.
- Wipe the skillet clean and add the remaining tablespoon of olive oil. Heat the skillet over medium heat.
- Pour the beaten eggs into the skillet and let them cook undisturbed for a minute or until the edges start to set.
- Gently lift the edges of the omelet with a spatula and tilt the skillet to allow the uncooked eggs to flow to the edges.
- Sprinkle the cooked vegetables, crumbled feta cheese, and chopped parsley evenly over one side of the omelet.
- Fold the other side of the omelet over the filling and press it gently with the spatula.
- Cook the omelet for another minute or until the eggs are fully cooked and the cheese has melted.

- Carefully slide the omelet onto a plate and cut it into wedges.
- Serve the Mediterranean omelet hot with a side of fresh salad or toasted bread.

Enjoy your delicious Mediterranean omelet!

Chapter 5: Lunch and Dinner Recipes

Baked Salmon with Lemon and Dill

Baked salmon with lemon and dill is a delicious and healthy dish that is easy to prepare. Here's a simple recipe to guide you:

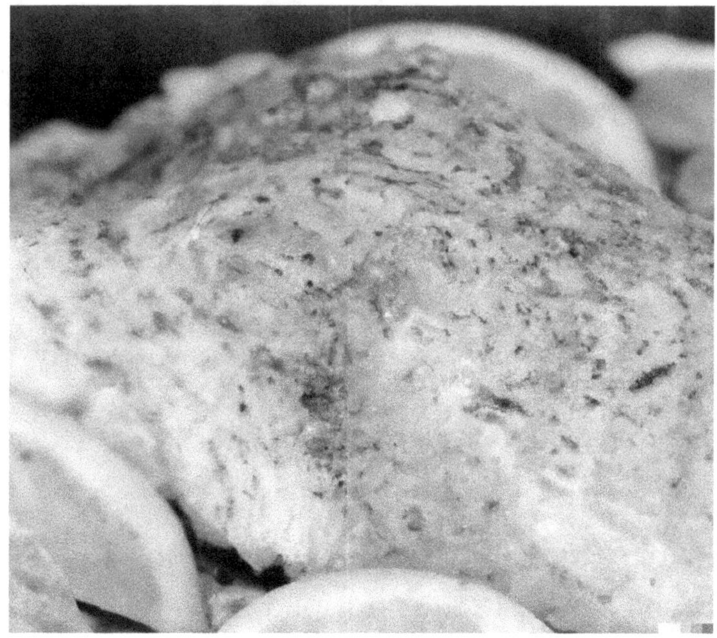

Ingredients:

- 1 pound salmon fillet
- 1 lemon
- Fresh dill, chopped
- Salt and pepper, to taste
- Olive oil

Instructions:

Preheat your oven to 375°F (190°C).

Place the salmon fillet on a baking dish lined with aluminum foil or parchment paper. This helps with easy cleanup later.

Squeeze the juice of half a lemon over the salmon fillet, ensuring the juice covers the entire surface.

Sprinkle salt and pepper over the salmon, according to your taste preferences. Be sure to season both sides of the fillet.

Take a handful of fresh dill and chop it finely. Sprinkle the chopped dill over the salmon, evenly distributing it.

Slice the remaining half of the lemon into thin rounds. Place the lemon slices on top of the salmon fillet.

Drizzle a small amount of olive oil over the salmon to keep it moist during baking.

Cover the baking dish with foil, creating a loose tent. This will help the salmon cook evenly and retain its moisture.

Place the baking dish in the preheated oven and bake for approximately 15-20 minutes, or until the salmon is cooked through and flakes easily with a fork. Cooking times may vary depending on the thickness of your fillet, so keep an eye on it.

Once the salmon is cooked, remove it from the oven and let it rest for a few minutes before serving.

Serve the baked salmon with lemon and dill alongside your favorite sides such as roasted vegetables, steamed rice, or a fresh salad. Enjoy!

Quinoa and Vegetable Stir-Fry

Quinoa and vegetable stir-fry is a delicious and healthy dish that combines the protein-rich quinoa with a colorful mix of vegetables. Here's a simple recipe to make quinoa and vegetable stir-fry:

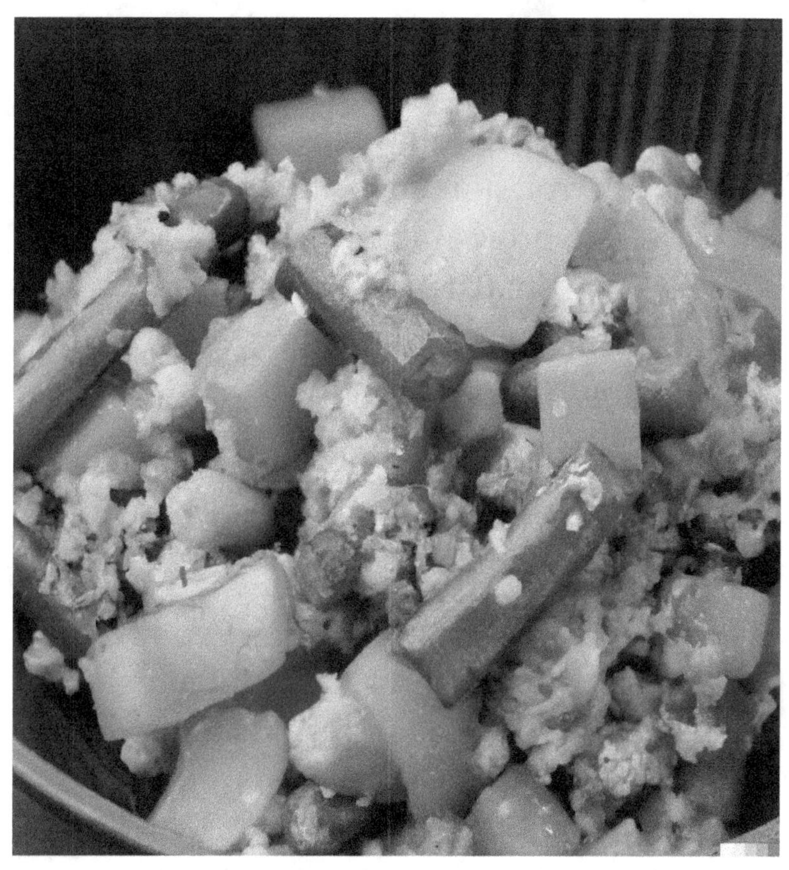

Ingredients:

- 1 cup quinoa
- 2 cups water
- 2 tablespoons olive oil
- 1 onion, thinly sliced
- 2 cloves garlic, minced

- 1 red bell pepper, thinly sliced
- 1 yellow bell pepper, thinly sliced
- 1 zucchini, thinly sliced
- 1 carrot, julienned
- 1 cup broccoli florets
- 1 cup snap peas
- 2 tablespoons soy sauce
- 1 tablespoon sesame oil
- Salt and pepper to taste
- Optional toppings: sesame seeds, chopped green onions

Instructions:

Rinse the quinoa thoroughly under cold water to remove any bitterness. In a saucepan, combine the rinsed quinoa and water. Bring to a boil, then reduce the heat to low, cover, and simmer for about 15-20 minutes or until the quinoa is cooked and the water is absorbed. Remove from heat and let it sit covered for 5 minutes. Fluff the quinoa with a fork and set aside.

In a large skillet or wok, heat the olive oil over medium heat. Add the onion and garlic, and sauté for 2-3 minutes until they become fragrant and slightly translucent.

Add the sliced bell peppers, zucchini, carrot, broccoli, and snap peas to the skillet. Stir-fry the vegetables for 5-7 minutes or until they are tender-crisp. You can adjust the cooking time based on your preference for the crunchiness of the vegetables.

In a small bowl, whisk together the soy sauce and sesame oil. Pour the mixture over the vegetables in the skillet and toss to coat evenly. Season with salt and pepper to taste.

Add the cooked quinoa to the skillet and stir-fry for an additional 2-3 minutes, allowing the flavors to blend together.

Remove the skillet from the heat and serve the quinoa and vegetable stir-fry hot.

Garnish with sesame seeds and chopped green onions if desired.

This recipe serves about 4-6 servings, depending on the portion size. Feel free to customize the stir-fry by adding or substituting other vegetables of your choice. Enjoy your nutritious quinoa and vegetable stir-fry!

Grilled Chicken Salad with Balsamic Dressing

Grilled Chicken Salad with Balsamic Dressing is a delicious and healthy dish that combines the flavors of tender grilled chicken, crisp vegetables, and a tangy balsamic dressing. Here's a recipe to guide you through the preparation:

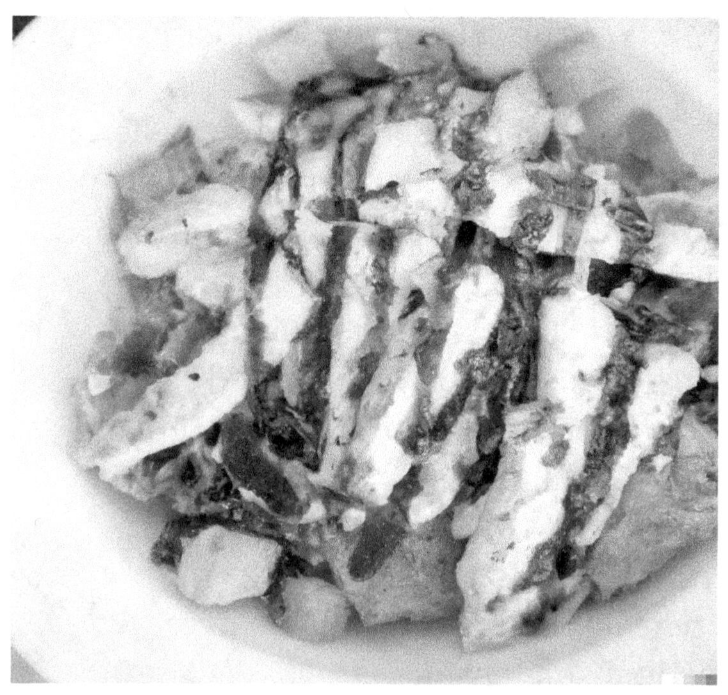

Ingredients:

For the salad:

- 2 boneless, skinless chicken breasts
- Salt and pepper, to taste
- 6 cups mixed salad greens (such as lettuce, spinach, or arugula)
- 1 cup cherry tomatoes, halved
- 1 cucumber, sliced
- 1/2 red onion, thinly sliced
- 1/4 cup sliced black olives

- 1/4 cup crumbled feta cheese (optional)
- 2 tablespoons chopped fresh herbs (such as basil or parsley)

For the balsamic dressing:
- 1/4 cup balsamic vinegar
- 1/4 cup extra virgin olive oil
- 1 teaspoon Dijon mustard
- 1 clove garlic, minced
- Salt and pepper, to taste

Instructions:

Preheat your grill or grill pan over medium-high heat.

Season the chicken breasts with salt and pepper on both sides. Grill the chicken for about 6-8 minutes per side, or until cooked through. Remove from the grill and let it rest for a few minutes. Once rested, slice the chicken into thin strips.

Meanwhile, prepare the salad by combining the mixed salad greens, cherry tomatoes, cucumber, red onion, black olives, and crumbled feta cheese (if using) in a large bowl. Toss to combine.

In a small bowl, whisk together the balsamic vinegar, olive oil, Dijon mustard, minced garlic, salt, and pepper until well combined. Adjust the seasoning to your taste.

Pour the balsamic dressing over the salad and toss to coat the ingredients evenly.

Divide the salad into individual serving plates or bowls. Top each serving with the grilled chicken slices and sprinkle with fresh herbs.

Serve the grilled chicken salad immediately and enjoy!

Feel free to customize this recipe by adding your favorite vegetables or toppings. You can also add toasted nuts, avocado slices, or croutons for extra flavor and texture. Enjoy your Grilled Chicken Salad with Balsamic Dressing!

Zucchini Noodles with Tomato Sauce

Zucchini noodles, also known as "zoodles," are a healthy and delicious alternative to traditional pasta. Paired with a flavorful tomato sauce, they make a satisfying and nutritious meal. Here's a simple recipe for zucchini noodles with tomato sauce:

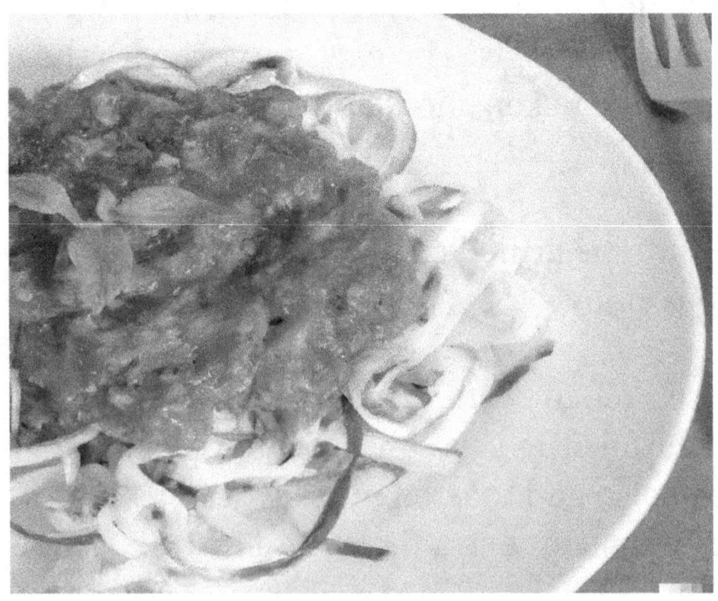

Ingredients:
- 2-3 large zucchini
- 2 tablespoons olive oil
- 2 cloves garlic, minced
- 1 can (14 ounces) diced tomatoes
- 1 can (6 ounces) tomato paste
- 1 teaspoon dried basil
- 1 teaspoon dried oregano
- Salt and pepper to taste
- Grated Parmesan cheese (optional)

Instructions:

Start by preparing the zucchini noodles. You can use a spiralizer to create long, spaghetti-like strands from the zucchini. If you don't have a spiralizer, you can use a julienne peeler or a sharp knife to slice the zucchini into thin, noodle-like strips. Set the zucchini noodles aside.

Heat the olive oil in a large skillet over medium heat. Add the minced garlic and sauté for about 1 minute until fragrant.

Add the diced tomatoes and tomato paste to the skillet, stirring well to combine. Season with dried basil, dried oregano, salt, and pepper. You can adjust the seasonings according to your taste preferences.

Bring the tomato sauce to a simmer and let it cook for about 10-15 minutes, allowing the flavors to meld together and the sauce to thicken slightly.

While the sauce is simmering, heat a separate skillet over medium heat. Add a little olive oil and the zucchini noodles. Sauté the noodles for about 2-3 minutes until they are just tender. Be careful not to overcook them, as they can become mushy.

Once the zucchini noodles are cooked, remove them from the heat and drain any excess liquid.

Divide the zucchini noodles onto serving plates or bowls. Top with a generous amount of the tomato sauce.

If desired, sprinkle grated Parmesan cheese over the zucchini noodles and tomato sauce.

Serve the zucchini noodles with tomato sauce immediately and enjoy!

This recipe is a healthy, low-carb alternative to traditional pasta dishes. It's a great way to incorporate more vegetables into your diet while still enjoying a delicious and satisfying meal. Feel free to customize the recipe by adding additional vegetables, such as sautéed mushrooms or spinach, or by garnishing with fresh herbs like basil or parsley.

Turkey Lettuce Wraps

Turkey lettuce wraps are a delicious and healthy dish that combines lean ground turkey with fresh vegetables and flavorful seasonings, all wrapped up in crisp lettuce leaves. Here's a simple recipe to guide you in making turkey lettuce wraps:

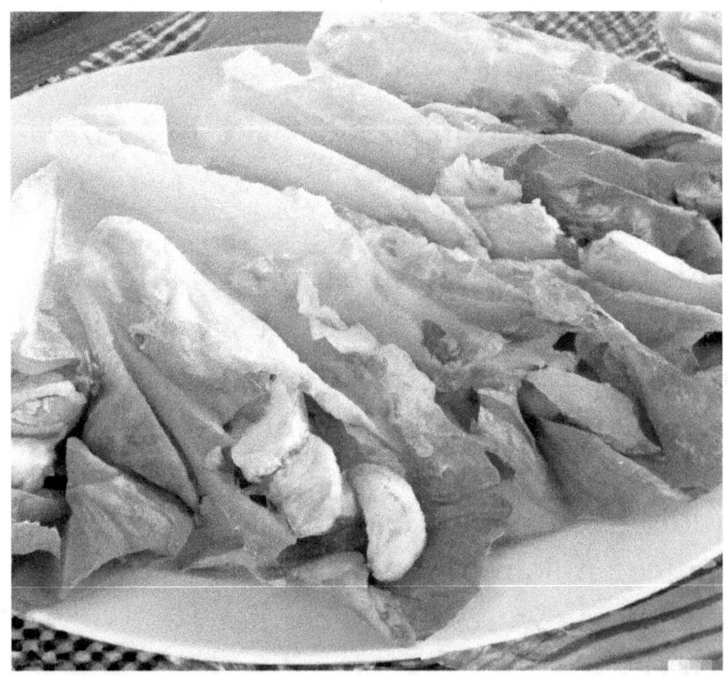

Ingredients:
- 1 lb (450g) ground turkey
- 2 tablespoons vegetable oil
- 2 cloves garlic, minced

- 1 small onion, finely chopped
- 1 red bell pepper, diced
- 1 carrot, shredded
- 1/4 cup hoisin sauce
- 2 tablespoons soy sauce
- 1 tablespoon rice vinegar
- 1 teaspoon sesame oil
- Salt and pepper to taste
- Lettuce leaves (such as iceberg or butter lettuce)

Optional toppings:
- Chopped green onions
- Chopped cilantro
- Chopped peanuts
- Sriracha or hot sauce

Instructions:
- Heat the vegetable oil in a large skillet or wok over medium-high heat.
- Add the minced garlic and chopped onion to the pan and sauté for 2-3 minutes until fragrant and slightly softened.

- Add the ground turkey to the pan, breaking it up with a spatula. Cook for about 5-6 minutes until the turkey is cooked through and no longer pink.
- Add the diced bell pepper and shredded carrot to the skillet. Cook for an additional 2-3 minutes until the vegetables are tender-crisp.
- In a small bowl, whisk together the hoisin sauce, soy sauce, rice vinegar, and sesame oil. Pour the sauce over the turkey and vegetables in the pan. Stir well to combine and coat everything evenly. Cook for another minute or two until the sauce is heated through.
- Taste the mixture and season with salt and pepper according to your preference.
- Remove the skillet from the heat and let the mixture cool slightly.
- Wash and dry the lettuce leaves, then use them as the wraps for the turkey mixture. Spoon a portion of the turkey

mixture into the center of each lettuce leaf.
- Add your desired toppings such as chopped green onions, cilantro, chopped peanuts, and a drizzle of sriracha or hot sauce.
- Serve the turkey lettuce wraps immediately and enjoy!

These turkey lettuce wraps are versatile, and you can customize them by adding or substituting other vegetables, herbs, or sauces based on your taste preferences. They make a great appetizer, light lunch, or even a healthy dinner option.

Chapter 6: Snacks and Appetizers

Kale Chips

Kale chips are a healthy and delicious snack made from kale leaves that have been baked or dehydrated until crispy. Kale, a nutrient-dense leafy green vegetable, is rich in vitamins A, C, and K, as well as minerals like calcium and potassium. It's also a good source of fiber.

To make kale chips, start by washing and drying the kale leaves thoroughly. Remove the tough stems and tear the leaves into bite-sized pieces. Preheat your oven to around 300°F (150°C).

Next, toss the kale pieces in a bowl with a small amount of olive oil or your preferred cooking oil. You want to coat the leaves evenly but not soak them. You can also add some seasonings like salt, pepper, garlic powder, or paprika for extra flavor.

Spread the kale pieces out in a single layer on a baking sheet lined with parchment paper. Make sure they aren't overcrowded to allow for even baking. Place the baking sheet in the preheated oven and bake for about 10-15 minutes, or until the kale chips turn crispy and slightly golden. Keep a close eye on them as they can burn quickly.

If you prefer a more hands-off approach, you can also use a food dehydrator to make kale chips. Simply arrange the oiled and seasoned kale pieces on the dehydrator trays and follow the manufacturer's instructions for drying time and temperature.

Once the kale chips are done, remove them from the oven or dehydrator and let them cool completely before enjoying. They should be crispy and have a delicate texture.

Store any leftovers in an airtight container to maintain their crispiness.

Kale chips are a nutritious alternative to traditional potato chips and make a great snack for those looking to incorporate more leafy greens into their diet. They're also customizable, so feel free to experiment with different seasonings and spices to suit your taste preferences.

Roasted Chickpeas

Roasted chickpeas are a delicious and healthy snack that can be enjoyed on their own or added to salads, soups, or as a crunchy topping for various dishes. Here's a simple recipe to make roasted chickpeas:

Ingredients:
- 2 cans of chickpeas (garbanzo beans), drained and rinsed
- 2 tablespoons of olive oil
- 1 teaspoon of salt

- 1 teaspoon of paprika
- 1/2 teaspoon of garlic powder
- 1/2 teaspoon of cumin (optional)
- Optional seasonings: chili powder, cayenne pepper, curry powder, or any other spices you like

Instructions:

Preheat your oven to 400°F (200°C).

Drain and rinse the chickpeas thoroughly. Pat them dry using a clean kitchen towel or paper towels. Removing excess moisture will help them get crispy during roasting.

In a bowl, combine the olive oil, salt, paprika, garlic powder, and any additional seasonings you'd like to use. Stir well to create a seasoning mixture.

Add the chickpeas to the bowl and toss them with the seasoning mixture until they are evenly coated.

Spread the chickpeas out in a single layer on a baking sheet. Make sure they are not crowded to ensure even cooking.

Place the baking sheet in the preheated oven and roast the chickpeas for about 25-30 minutes, or until they are golden brown and crispy. It's a good idea to give them a shake or stir halfway through to ensure even browning.

Once roasted, remove the chickpeas from the oven and let them cool on the baking sheet for a few minutes. They will become even crispier as they cool down.

Enjoy the roasted chickpeas as a snack or use them in your favorite recipes!

Roasted chickpeas can be stored in an airtight container at room temperature for a few days. However, note that they may lose some of their crispiness over time.

Guacamole with Veggie Sticks

Guacamole with veggie sticks is a delicious and healthy snack or appetizer option. Guacamole is a popular Mexican dip made from mashed avocados, combined with various ingredients for flavor. Veggie sticks, such as carrot sticks, celery sticks, bell pepper strips, or cucumber slices, are perfect for dipping into the creamy guacamole. Here's a simple recipe to make guacamole and serve it with veggie sticks:

Ingredients:

- 2 ripe avocados
- 1 small onion, finely chopped
- 1 small tomato, diced
- 1-2 cloves of garlic, minced
- 1 jalapeño pepper, seeded and minced (optional, for some heat)
- Juice of 1 lime
- 2 tablespoons chopped fresh cilantro (coriander)
- Salt and pepper to taste

- Assorted veggie sticks for dipping
  (carrots, celery, bell peppers,
  cucumbers, etc.)

Instructions:

- Cut the avocados in half lengthwise
  and remove the pits. Scoop out the
  flesh into a bowl.
- Mash the avocados using a fork until
  you achieve your desired
  consistency—some prefer it smooth,
  while others like it chunky.
- Add the finely chopped onion, diced
  tomato, minced garlic, and minced
  jalapeño pepper (if using) to the
  mashed avocados.
- Squeeze the juice of one lime into the
  bowl to prevent the avocados from
  browning and to add a tangy flavor.
- Add the chopped cilantro to the
  mixture. You can adjust the amount
  based on your preference for cilantro.

- Season the guacamole with salt and pepper to taste. Stir all the ingredients together until well combined.
- Taste the guacamole and adjust the seasoning or add more lime juice if needed.
- Transfer the guacamole to a serving bowl and place it in the center of a platter.
- Arrange the assorted veggie sticks around the guacamole bowl.
- Serve the guacamole with the veggie sticks and enjoy!

Feel free to customize the recipe based on your taste preferences. You can add additional ingredients like diced bell peppers, corn, or black beans to the guacamole for extra flavor and texture. Enjoy your guacamole with veggie sticks as a healthy snack or as part of a party spread.

Spicy Oven-Baked Sweet Potato Fries

Spicy oven-baked sweet potato fries are a delicious and healthy alternative to traditional French fries. Here's a simple recipe to make them:

Ingredients:
- 2 large sweet potatoes
- 2 tablespoons olive oil
- 1 teaspoon paprika
- 1/2 teaspoon chili powder
- 1/2 teaspoon garlic powder
- 1/2 teaspoon salt
- 1/4 teaspoon black pepper

Instructions:
- Preheat your oven to 425°F (220°C) and line a baking sheet with parchment paper or foil.
- Wash and peel the sweet potatoes. Cut them into thin, even-sized strips, resembling the shape of fries.

- In a large bowl, combine the olive oil, paprika, chili powder, garlic powder, salt, and black pepper. Mix well.
- Add the sweet potato strips to the bowl and toss them in the spice mixture until evenly coated.
- Arrange the coated sweet potato strips in a single layer on the prepared baking sheet, making sure they're not crowded. This will help them crisp up.
- Place the baking sheet in the preheated oven and bake for about 25-30 minutes, flipping the fries halfway through. Bake until the fries are crispy and golden brown.
- Once baked, remove the fries from the oven and let them cool for a few minutes before serving. This will help them get even crispier.
- Serve the spicy oven-baked sweet potato fries as a side dish or a snack. They're great on their own or paired with your favorite dipping sauce.

Enjoy your homemade spicy oven-baked sweet potato fries!

Greek Yogurt and Berry Parfait

A Greek yogurt and berry parfait is a delicious and healthy layered dessert or breakfast option that combines creamy Greek yogurt with fresh berries and other toppings. It's easy to prepare and can be customized with your favorite fruits, nuts, and sweeteners. Here's a simple recipe to make a Greek yogurt and berry parfait:

Ingredients:
- 1 cup Greek yogurt
- 1 cup mixed berries (such as strawberries, blueberries, raspberries)
- 1/4 cup granola or crushed nuts
- Honey or maple syrup (optional, for added sweetness)

Instructions:

- Wash and prepare the berries by slicing any large fruits like strawberries.
- In a clear glass or parfait dish, start by adding a layer of Greek yogurt at the bottom.
- Add a layer of mixed berries on top of the yogurt.
- Sprinkle a layer of granola or crushed nuts over the berries.
- Repeat the layers until you've used up all the ingredients or reached your desired amount.
- Drizzle honey or maple syrup on top if you prefer a sweeter parfait.
- Finish with a final sprinkle of granola or nuts for added texture and presentation.
- Serve immediately and enjoy!

Feel free to experiment with different variations by adding other fruits, seeds, or even a dollop of nut butter. You can also prepare the parfaits in advance and refrigerate them for a few hours to let the flavors meld together. Just be sure to add any crunchy toppings just before serving to maintain their texture. Enjoy your Greek yogurt and berry parfait!

Chapter 7: Soups and Stews

Lentil Soup with Vegetables

Ingredients:

- 1 cup dried lentils (green or brown), rinsed and drained
- 1 tablespoon olive oil
- 1 onion, diced
- 2 cloves garlic, minced
- 2 carrots, diced
- 2 celery stalks, diced
- 1 bell pepper, diced (any color you prefer)
- 1 zucchini, diced
- 4 cups vegetable broth
- 1 can (14 oz) diced tomatoes
- 1 teaspoon dried thyme
- 1 teaspoon dried oregano
- 1 bay leaf
- Salt and pepper to taste
- Fresh parsley, chopped (for garnish)

Instructions:

- Heat the olive oil in a large pot or Dutch oven over medium heat.
- Add the diced onion and minced garlic to the pot and sauté until the onion becomes translucent and fragrant.
- Add the diced carrots, celery, bell pepper, and zucchini to the pot. Sauté for about 5 minutes, until the vegetables start to soften.
- Add the rinsed lentils, vegetable broth, diced tomatoes (including the juice), dried thyme, dried oregano, and bay leaf to the pot. Stir well to combine.
- Bring the soup to a boil, then reduce the heat to low. Cover the pot and let it simmer for about 30-40 minutes, or until the lentils are tender and cooked through.
- Season with salt and pepper to taste. Remove the bay leaf from the pot.
- Serve the lentil soup hot, garnished with fresh parsley.

Enjoy your homemade Lentil Soup with Vegetables! It's a hearty and nutritious dish that's perfect for a comforting meal.

Chicken and Vegetable Soup

Chicken and vegetable soup is a delicious and nutritious dish that combines the flavors of tender chicken with a medley of fresh vegetables. It's a comforting and satisfying meal that can be enjoyed any time of the year. Here's a basic recipe to get you started:

Ingredients:
- 1 pound (450g) boneless, skinless chicken breasts or thighs, diced
- 1 tablespoon olive oil
- 1 onion, diced
- 2 cloves of garlic, minced
- 2 carrots, sliced
- 2 celery stalks, sliced
- 1 zucchini, diced

- 1 cup corn kernels (fresh or frozen)
- 4 cups chicken broth
- 2 cups water
- 1 teaspoon dried thyme
- 1 teaspoon dried oregano
- Salt and pepper to taste
- Fresh parsley or cilantro for garnish (optional)

Instructions:
Heat the olive oil in a large pot or Dutch oven over medium heat. Add the diced chicken and cook until browned on all sides. Remove the chicken from the pot and set aside.

In the same pot, add the diced onion and minced garlic. Sauté for a few minutes until the onion becomes translucent and fragrant.

Add the sliced carrots, celery, zucchini, and corn to the pot. Stir and cook for another 5 minutes to soften the vegetables slightly.

Return the browned chicken to the pot and pour in the chicken broth and water. Add the dried thyme and oregano, and season with salt and pepper to taste. Bring the soup to a boil.

Once the soup reaches a boil, reduce the heat to low and let it simmer for about 20-25 minutes, or until the chicken is cooked through and the vegetables are tender.

Taste the soup and adjust the seasoning if needed. You can add more salt, pepper, or herbs according to your preference.

Ladle the chicken and vegetable soup into bowls and garnish with fresh parsley or cilantro if desired. Serve hot and enjoy!

Butternut Squash and Apple Soup

Butternut squash and apple soup is a delicious and comforting dish that combines the natural sweetness of butternut squash with the tartness of apples. Here's a simple recipe to make this flavorful soup:

Ingredients:
- 1 medium-sized butternut squash
- 2 apples (such as Granny Smith or Fuji)
- 1 medium onion, chopped
- 2 cloves of garlic, minced
- 4 cups vegetable or chicken broth
- 1/2 teaspoon ground cinnamon
- 1/4 teaspoon ground nutmeg
- 1/4 teaspoon ground ginger
- Salt and pepper to taste
- 2 tablespoons olive oil
- Optional toppings: toasted pumpkin seeds, sour cream, or chopped fresh herbs (such as parsley or thyme)

Instructions:
Preheat your oven to 400°F (200°C). Cut the butternut squash in half lengthwise and remove the seeds. Place the squash halves on a baking sheet, cut side up. Drizzle with 1

tablespoon of olive oil and sprinkle with salt and pepper. Roast in the oven for about 40-45 minutes or until the flesh is tender and easily pierced with a fork.

While the squash is roasting, peel, core, and chop the apples into small pieces.

In a large pot, heat the remaining 1 tablespoon of olive oil over medium heat. Add the chopped onion and minced garlic, and sauté until they become soft and translucent, about 5 minutes.

Add the chopped apples to the pot and cook for an additional 5 minutes, stirring occasionally.

Once the roasted butternut squash is done, let it cool slightly, then scoop out the flesh and add it to the pot with the onion, garlic, and apples. Discard the skin.

Stir in the ground cinnamon, nutmeg, ginger, salt, and pepper. Pour in the vegetable or chicken broth and bring the mixture to a boil.

Reduce the heat to low and simmer the soup for about 15-20 minutes to allow the flavors to blend together.

Use an immersion blender or transfer the soup in batches to a blender, and blend until smooth and creamy. Be careful when blending hot liquids to prevent any accidents.

Return the soup to the pot and adjust the seasoning if needed. If the soup is too thick, you can add a little more broth or water to reach the desired consistency.

Reheat the soup over low heat if necessary before serving. Ladle the soup into bowls and garnish with optional toppings like toasted pumpkin seeds, a dollop of sour cream, or chopped fresh herbs.

Enjoy your delicious butternut squash and apple soup! It pairs well with crusty bread or a side salad for a complete meal.

Beef and Barley Stew

Ingredients:
- 1.5 pounds (680g) beef stew meat, cut into bite-sized pieces
- 1 tablespoon vegetable oil
- 1 large onion, diced
- 2 carrots, diced
- 2 celery stalks, diced
- 3 cloves of garlic, minced
- 6 cups beef broth
- 1 cup water
- 1 cup pearl barley
- 2 bay leaves
- 1 teaspoon dried thyme
- Salt and pepper to taste

- Chopped fresh parsley for garnish
  (optional)

Instructions:
- Heat the vegetable oil in a large pot or
  Dutch oven over medium-high heat.
- Add the beef stew meat to the pot and
  brown it on all sides. This will add
  flavor to the stew. Once browned,
  remove the beef from the pot and set it
  aside.
- In the same pot, add the diced onion,
  carrots, celery, and minced garlic.
  Sauté the vegetables until they begin
  to soften, about 5 minutes.
- Return the browned beef to the pot
  with the vegetables.
- Add the beef broth, water, pearl
  barley, bay leaves, and dried thyme to
  the pot. Stir everything together.
- Bring the stew to a boil, then reduce
  the heat to low and cover the pot.
  Simmer the stew for about 1 to 1.5
  hours, or until the beef is tender and

the barley is cooked through. Stir
occasionally.

- Season the stew with salt and pepper
to taste. Remove the bay leaves before
serving.
- Ladle the beef and barley stew into
bowls and garnish with chopped fresh
parsley if desired.

Enjoy your hearty beef and barley stew! It
pairs well with crusty bread or a side salad.

Creamy Cauliflower Soup

Creamy cauliflower soup is a delicious and
nutritious dish that can be enjoyed as a
starter or a light meal. Here's a simple
recipe to make creamy cauliflower soup:

Ingredients:
- 1 large cauliflower, chopped into
florets
- 1 onion, chopped
- 2 cloves of garlic, minced

- 4 cups vegetable or chicken broth
- 1 cup milk or cream (you can use almond milk or coconut milk as a dairy-free alternative)
- 2 tablespoons butter or olive oil
- Salt and pepper to taste
- Optional toppings: grated cheese, chopped fresh herbs, croutons, or a drizzle of olive oil

Instructions:

In a large pot, melt the butter or heat the olive oil over medium heat. Add the chopped onion and minced garlic and sauté until they become soft and translucent.

Add the cauliflower florets to the pot and stir them with the onions and garlic. Season with salt and pepper to taste.

Pour in the vegetable or chicken broth, making sure the cauliflower is fully covered. Bring the mixture to a boil, then reduce the heat to low and let it simmer for about 15-20 minutes or until the cauliflower is tender.

Once the cauliflower is cooked, remove the pot from the heat and let it cool slightly. Using an immersion blender or a regular blender, puree the soup until smooth and creamy. Be careful when blending hot liquids, and you may need to do it in batches if using a regular blender.

Return the pureed soup to the pot and place it back on the stove over low heat. Stir in the milk or cream and heat the soup until warmed through, but do not let it boil.

Taste the soup and adjust the seasoning if needed.

Serve the creamy cauliflower soup hot, garnished with your desired toppings such as grated cheese, chopped fresh herbs, croutons, or a drizzle of olive oil.

Chapter 8: Side Dishes

Quinoa Pilaf

Quinoa pilaf is a delicious and nutritious dish made with quinoa, a grain-like seed that is rich in protein and fiber. Pilaf is a cooking method where the grain is first toasted in oil or butter before being cooked in liquid, resulting in a flavorful and fluffy dish. Here's a basic recipe for quinoa pilaf:

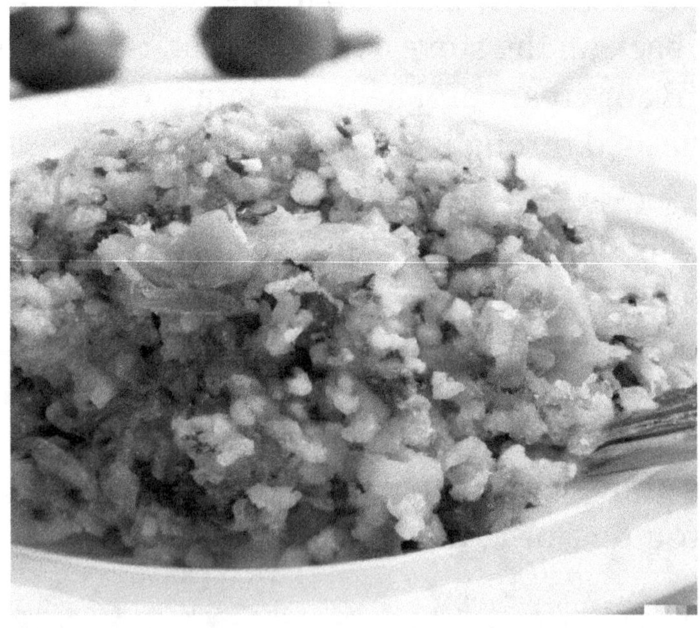

Ingredients:

- 1 cup quinoa
- 2 cups vegetable or chicken broth
- 1 tablespoon olive oil or butter
- 1 small onion, finely chopped
- 2 cloves garlic, minced
- 1/2 cup chopped vegetables (such as carrots, bell peppers, or peas)
- Salt and pepper to taste
- Optional: herbs and spices of your choice (such as thyme, cumin, or paprika)

Instructions:

- Rinse the quinoa thoroughly in a fine-mesh strainer to remove any bitterness.
- Heat the olive oil or butter in a large saucepan over medium heat.
- Add the chopped onion and sauté for about 5 minutes until it becomes translucent.

- Add the minced garlic and chopped vegetables to the pan and cook for an additional 2-3 minutes.
- Add the rinsed quinoa to the pan and stir to combine it with the vegetables. Cook for 1-2 minutes to lightly toast the quinoa.
- Pour in the vegetable or chicken broth and season with salt, pepper, and any additional herbs or spices you desire.
- Bring the mixture to a boil, then reduce the heat to low and cover the saucepan with a lid.
- Let the quinoa simmer for about 15-20 minutes or until all the liquid has been absorbed and the quinoa is tender.
- Remove the saucepan from the heat and let it sit, covered, for an additional 5 minutes to allow the quinoa to fluff up.
- Fluff the quinoa pilaf with a fork and serve it hot as a side dish or as a base for your favorite protein or vegetable toppings.

Feel free to customize the quinoa pilaf by adding other ingredients like nuts, dried fruits, or fresh herbs. Enjoy your flavorful and nutritious quinoa pilaf!

Roasted Brussels Sprouts with Balsamic Glaze

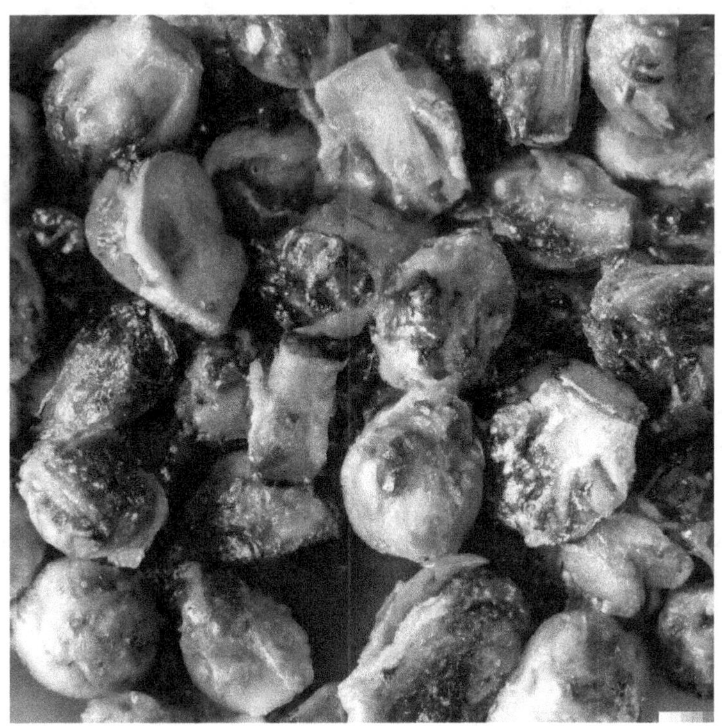

Ingredients:

- 1 pound Brussels sprouts
- 2 tablespoons olive oil
- Salt and pepper to taste
- 2 tablespoons balsamic vinegar
- 1 tablespoon honey or maple syrup (optional, for added sweetness)

Instructions:

Preheat your oven to 425°F (220°C).

Rinse the Brussels sprouts under cold water and trim off any tough outer leaves. Cut off the stem end of each sprout and then cut them in half.

Place the halved Brussels sprouts in a large mixing bowl and drizzle with olive oil. Toss them well to ensure even coating.

Season the sprouts with salt and pepper according to your taste. You can also add other seasonings like garlic powder or dried herbs if desired.

Spread the Brussels sprouts out in a single layer on a baking sheet. Make sure they're not too crowded to allow even roasting.

Place the baking sheet in the preheated oven and roast for about 20-25 minutes, or until the sprouts are tender and slightly caramelized. You can give them a gentle stir halfway through cooking for more even browning.

While the Brussels sprouts are roasting, prepare the balsamic glaze. In a small saucepan, combine the balsamic vinegar and honey (or maple syrup) over medium heat. Bring the mixture to a simmer, stirring occasionally.

Allow the balsamic glaze to simmer for about 5-7 minutes, or until it thickens slightly and coats the back of a spoon.

Remove the saucepan from heat and set aside.

Once the Brussels sprouts are roasted, remove them from the oven and transfer to a serving dish.

Drizzle the balsamic glaze over the roasted Brussels sprouts, tossing gently to coat them evenly.

Serve the roasted Brussels sprouts with balsamic glaze immediately as a side dish or as a tasty appetizer.

Enjoy your delicious roasted Brussels sprouts with balsamic glaze

Steamed Broccoli with Garlic

Steamed broccoli with garlic is a simple and delicious way to prepare this nutritious vegetable. Here's a basic recipe to guide you:

Ingredients:

- 1 head of broccoli
- 2 cloves of garlic, minced
- 2 tablespoons olive oil
- Salt and pepper to taste

Instructions:

Start by preparing the broccoli. Cut off the florets from the head of broccoli, leaving them in bite-sized pieces. You can also peel the tough outer skin of the stem and slice it into thin rounds if desired.

Fill a pot with about an inch of water and bring it to a boil. Place a steamer basket or colander over the pot, making sure it doesn't touch the water. Add the broccoli florets and stems to the steamer basket.

Cover the pot with a lid and steam the broccoli for about 5-7 minutes or until it becomes bright green and tender. Be careful not to overcook it, as you want the broccoli to maintain some crunch.

While the broccoli is steaming, heat the olive oil in a small pan over medium heat. Add the minced garlic and sauté for about a minute until it becomes fragrant and lightly golden. Remove the pan from heat.

Once the broccoli is steamed, transfer it to a serving bowl. Drizzle the garlic-infused olive oil over the broccoli, making sure to distribute it evenly. Toss the broccoli gently to coat it with the oil and garlic.

Season with salt and pepper to taste. You can also squeeze some lemon juice over the steamed broccoli for a refreshing twist, if desired.

Serve the steamed broccoli with garlic as a side dish alongside your favorite main course. It pairs well with grilled chicken, fish, or even as a topping for pasta or salads.

Enjoy your steamed broccoli with garlic! It's a nutritious and flavorful addition to any meal.

Cucumber and Tomato Salad

Cucumber and tomato salad is a refreshing and simple dish that is perfect for summer or as a side dish with various meals. Here's a basic recipe to get you started:

Ingredients:
- 2 medium-sized cucumbers
- 4 medium-sized tomatoes
- 1 small red onion
- 1/4 cup fresh parsley, chopped
- 2 tablespoons fresh dill, chopped
- 2 tablespoons extra virgin olive oil
- 1 tablespoon lemon juice (optional)
- Salt and pepper to taste

Instructions:
Wash the cucumbers and tomatoes thoroughly. You can peel the cucumbers if

desired, but it's not necessary. Slice the cucumbers and tomatoes into bite-sized pieces. You can choose to keep the skin on the tomatoes or remove it, depending on your preference.

Peel and thinly slice the red onion.

In a large bowl, combine the cucumber slices, tomato slices, and sliced red onion.

Add the chopped parsley and dill to the bowl.

Drizzle the olive oil over the salad. If desired, squeeze fresh lemon juice over the salad for a tangy flavor.

Season with salt and pepper according to your taste. Toss the salad gently to ensure the ingredients are evenly coated with the dressing.

Let the salad sit for a few minutes to allow the flavors to meld together. You can also refrigerate it for about 30 minutes to chill before serving.

Serve the cucumber and tomato salad as a side dish or as a light and refreshing meal on its own.

Feel free to customize the salad by adding other ingredients such as feta cheese, olives, or avocado to suit your taste preferences. Enjoy!

Mashed Cauliflower

Mashed cauliflower is a healthy and flavorful alternative to traditional mashed potatoes. It is a dish made by boiling or steaming cauliflower until it becomes soft, then mashing it to a desired consistency. Here's a basic recipe for making mashed cauliflower:

Ingredients:

- 1 large head of cauliflower
- 2-3 cloves of garlic, minced (optional)
- 2 tablespoons butter or olive oil
- Salt and pepper to taste
- Fresh herbs for garnish (optional)

Instructions:

- Cut the cauliflower into florets, discarding the tough stem and leaves. Rinse the florets thoroughly.
- Bring a large pot of water to a boil and add the cauliflower florets. Cook for about 10-15 minutes, or until the cauliflower is tender and easily mashed with a fork.
- Drain the cauliflower and transfer it to a large mixing bowl.
- Add minced garlic, butter or olive oil, salt, and pepper to the bowl with the cauliflower.
- Mash the cauliflower using a potato masher or an immersion blender until it reaches your desired consistency. If

you prefer a smoother texture, you can also use a food processor.

- Taste and adjust the seasonings as needed.
- Transfer the mashed cauliflower to a serving dish and garnish with fresh herbs, if desired.
- Serve hot and enjoy as a side dish or as a healthier alternative to mashed potatoes.

You can also experiment with different flavors by adding grated cheese, chopped herbs, or spices such as paprika or nutmeg. Mashed cauliflower is a versatile dish that can be customized to your taste preferences.

Chapter 9: Desserts and Treats

Sugar-Free Chocolate Avocado Mousse

Ingredients:
- 2 ripe avocados
- 1/4 cup unsweetened cocoa powder
- 1/4 cup sugar-free sweetener (such as stevia or erythritol)
- 1/4 cup unsweetened almond milk (or any other non-dairy milk)
- 1 teaspoon vanilla extract
- Pinch of salt

Instructions:
- Cut the avocados in half, remove the pits, and scoop out the flesh into a blender or food processor.
- Add the cocoa powder, sugar-free sweetener, almond milk, vanilla extract, and salt to the blender or food processor.

- Blend until the mixture is smooth and creamy, scraping down the sides as needed.
- Taste the mousse and adjust the sweetness or cocoa powder to your liking.
- Transfer the mousse to serving glasses or bowls.
- Place the mousse in the refrigerator and chill for at least 1 hour to allow it to set.
- Serve chilled and enjoy!

This sugar-free chocolate avocado mousse is a healthier alternative to traditional chocolate mousse, as it doesn't contain added sugar. The natural sweetness of the ripe avocados, combined with the cocoa powder and sugar-free sweetener, creates a rich and creamy dessert that satisfies chocolate cravings without the guilt.

Berry Chia Seed Jam

Berry Chia Seed Jam is a delicious and nutritious alternative to traditional jam. It is made by combining fresh or frozen berries with chia seeds, which act as a natural thickening agent. The chia seeds absorb the liquid from the berries and create a gel-like consistency similar to jam. This recipe is simple, healthy, and doesn't require any added sugars or artificial preservatives. Here's a basic recipe to make your own Berry Chia Seed Jam:

Ingredients:

- 2 cups fresh or frozen berries (strawberries, blueberries, raspberries, or a combination)
- 2 tablespoons chia seeds
- 1 tablespoon lemon juice (optional, for added flavor)
- Sweetener of your choice (optional, if needed)

Instructions:

In a saucepan, add the berries and cook over medium heat until they soften and release their juices. If using frozen berries, you may need to add a splash of water to help them thaw and break down.

Once the berries have softened, use a potato masher or a fork to mash them until they reach your desired consistency. If you prefer a smoother jam, you can also use a blender or food processor.

Stir in the chia seeds and lemon juice (if using) into the mashed berries. Mix well to ensure the chia seeds are evenly distributed.

Let the mixture sit for about 10-15 minutes, stirring occasionally. This allows the chia seeds to absorb the liquid and thicken the jam.

Taste the jam and if you prefer it sweeter, you can add a sweetener of your choice such as honey, maple syrup, or stevia. Start with a small amount and adjust to your desired level of sweetness.

Once the jam has thickened to your liking, remove it from the heat and let it cool completely.

Transfer the jam to a jar or airtight container and refrigerate for at least a few hours or overnight. The jam will continue to thicken as it cools.

Enjoy your homemade Berry Chia Seed Jam on toast, pancakes, oatmeal, yogurt, or as a topping for desserts. It can be stored in the refrigerator for about 1-2 weeks.

Baked Apple with Cinnamon

Baked apples with cinnamon are a delicious and comforting dessert that is easy to make. Here's a simple recipe for baked apples with cinnamon:

Ingredients:

- 4 medium-sized apples (such as Granny Smith or Honeycrisp)
- 2 tablespoons unsalted butter, melted
- 2 tablespoons brown sugar
- 1 teaspoon ground cinnamon
- 1/4 teaspoon ground nutmeg (optional)
- 1/4 cup chopped nuts (such as walnuts or pecans)
- 1/4 cup raisins or dried cranberries (optional)
- Vanilla ice cream or whipped cream for serving (optional)

Instructions:

- Preheat your oven to 375°F (190°C).
- Wash the apples thoroughly and remove the cores, either by using an apple corer or by carefully cutting around the core with a sharp knife. Make sure to leave the bottom intact, creating a well for the filling.

- In a small bowl, mix together the melted butter, brown sugar, cinnamon, and nutmeg (if using).
- Place the apples in a baking dish or a lined baking sheet, and spoon the butter mixture into the well of each apple, dividing it evenly among them.
- Sprinkle the chopped nuts and raisins or dried cranberries (if using) over the top of each apple.
- Bake the apples in the preheated oven for about 30-35 minutes or until they are tender but not mushy. You can test their doneness by inserting a fork or toothpick into the flesh. It should slide in easily.
- Remove the baked apples from the oven and let them cool for a few minutes before serving.
- Serve the baked apples warm, either on their own or with a scoop of vanilla ice cream or a dollop of whipped cream for added indulgence.

Enjoy your delicious baked apples with cinnamon! They are perfect for a cozy dessert or a sweet treat any time of the year.

Coconut Flour Banana Bread

Ingredients:

- 4 ripe bananas
- 6 large eggs
- 1/2 cup coconut flour
- 1/4 cup coconut oil, melted
- 1/4 cup honey or maple syrup (optional, for sweetness)
- 1 teaspoon vanilla extract
- 1 teaspoon baking powder
- 1/2 teaspoon cinnamon
- 1/4 teaspoon salt

Instructions:

- Preheat your oven to 350°F (175°C). Grease a loaf pan with coconut oil or line it with parchment paper.
- In a mixing bowl, mash the ripe bananas until smooth.

- Add the eggs, melted coconut oil, honey or maple syrup (if using), and vanilla extract to the mashed bananas. Whisk together until well combined.
- In a separate bowl, combine the coconut flour, baking powder, cinnamon, and salt.
- Gradually add the dry ingredients to the wet ingredients, stirring well after each addition. Mix until you have a smooth batter without any lumps.
- Pour the batter into the greased or lined loaf pan, spreading it evenly.
- Bake in the preheated oven for about 50-60 minutes, or until a toothpick inserted into the center comes out clean.
- Remove the banana bread from the oven and let it cool in the pan for about 10 minutes. Then transfer it to a wire rack to cool completely before slicing.

Enjoy your homemade coconut flour banana bread!

Greek Yogurt with Fresh Berries

Greek yogurt with fresh berries is a delicious and nutritious combination that makes for a perfect breakfast, snack, or even a light dessert. Here's a simple recipe to enjoy this delightful treat:

Ingredients:
- 1 cup of Greek yogurt
- Fresh berries (such as strawberries, blueberries, raspberries, or blackberries)
- Honey or maple syrup (optional, for sweetening)

Instructions:
- Start by washing the fresh berries thoroughly under cold water and patting them dry with a paper towel.

- If the berries are large, you can chop them into smaller pieces or leave them whole, depending on your preference.
- Take a serving bowl or a glass and spoon in the Greek yogurt, filling it about halfway.
- Add a generous amount of fresh berries on top of the yogurt.
- If you prefer a touch of sweetness, drizzle some honey or maple syrup over the berries.
- You can garnish the yogurt and berries with a sprinkle of granola, nuts, or chia seeds for added texture and crunch, if desired.
- Gently mix everything together, ensuring that the yogurt and berries are well combined.
- Serve and enjoy your Greek yogurt with fresh berries immediately.

Conclusion

The Blood Sugar Diet offers a multitude of unique and comprehensive benefits that make it a powerful tool for improving health and well-being. By focusing on reducing refined sugars and carbohydrates while promoting nutrient-dense whole foods, this diet aims to regulate blood sugar levels and support weight loss.

One of the significant advantages of the Blood Sugar Diet is its ability to effectively address insulin resistance and manage blood sugar levels. By restricting the consumption of sugar and refined carbohydrates, the diet helps to stabilize blood glucose, preventing spikes and crashes that can lead to various health issues, including diabetes and metabolic syndrome. This stability in blood sugar levels promotes overall health and reduces the risk of chronic diseases.

Another notable benefit is the diet's positive impact on weight loss. By adopting a low-carbohydrate and low-calorie approach, the Blood Sugar Diet encourages the body to burn fat for energy instead of relying on glucose. This metabolic shift can result in significant weight loss, particularly around the abdominal area, which is crucial for reducing the risk of obesity-related complications such as heart disease and type 2 diabetes.

The Blood Sugar Diet also emphasizes the consumption of nutrient-dense whole foods, such as lean proteins, fruits, vegetables, and healthy fats. These food choices provide essential vitamins, minerals, and antioxidants that support overall health, boost the immune system, and reduce inflammation. Additionally, the diet encourages the consumption of high-fiber foods, which aids digestion, promotes satiety, and supports a healthy gut microbiome.

Moreover, the Blood Sugar Diet offers benefits beyond weight loss and blood sugar regulation. It has been associated with improved energy levels, increased mental clarity, enhanced mood, and better sleep quality. These effects can be attributed to the stable blood sugar levels achieved through the diet and the provision of essential nutrients that support overall physiological functioning.

Furthermore, the Blood Sugar Diet promotes healthier eating habits and encourages individuals to become more mindful of their food choices. By focusing on whole, unprocessed foods and limiting added sugars, it helps individuals break free from the cycle of craving and overconsumption of unhealthy foods. This can lead to a long-lasting positive change in eating behaviors and promote a sustainable approach to maintaining a healthy weight and overall well-being.

It is important to note that before starting any diet, including the Blood Sugar Diet, it is advisable to consult with a healthcare professional or registered dietitian to ensure it is appropriate for individual needs and medical conditions.